Coconut Oil For Hair
50 DIY Homemade Coconut Oil Hair Ma
By Ashley Frank

Printed In The United States of America

ISBN-13: 978-1514669365
ISBN-10: 1514669366

Cover photo design by Angie
Cover photos by DepositPhotos.com

Table of Contents

The History of Coconut Oil

Coconuts are said to have been discovered by early Spanish explorers in the tropical climates of islands in the Pacific. The explorers chose the name for this strange vegetation, choosing "coco", which means "monkey face", to describe the hairy-looking orb's appearance, and "nut" to denote that it comes from a nut bearing tree. It is not actually a nut, despite its name, but is related to olives and dates and is a "drupe". Coconuts thrive along coastlines and favor sandy soil. Thanks to seafarers and the fact that coconuts float, the drupe has spread far and wide. It is currently grown in 70+ countries. Major producers include India, Indonesia, Sri Lanka, and The Philippines.

The islanders that inhabited these warm Pacific regions when the Spanish explorers arrived were already familiar with the coconut's myriad of uses. These people relied on its plenitude for so many things that they called it, simply, "The Tree of Life". Coconuts provided nutrition when consumed in various delicious ways, but the islanders also relied on its medicinal powers to treat everything from asthma to typhoid to menstrual cramps. Coconut oil is still widely used in modern medicine because of its unique composition.

The oil is made up of around 90% saturated fat, 6% monounsaturated fat, and 3% polyunsaturated fat. It is different from other highly saturated and unsaturated fats because it is made up of medium chain fatty-acids. MCFA's are easier for the human body to break down and offer a huge number of health benefits including giving metabolism a boost. Coconut oil is also full of Lauric acid, a substance that is also found in human breast milk. Lauric acid is a natural antiviral, anti-fungal, and antibacterial agent.

Furthermore, the liquid found inside a coconut is very similar to the fluids found in human cells. It is full of electrolytes, natural sugars, and essential amino acids. So perfectly compatible with the human body was this coconut water that it was used in the I.V.'s of soldiers during World War II straight from a hole in the shell.

How is Coconut Oil Made?

The elixir that aids human beings in so many ways is found in the meat of the coconut. Modern advancements have created ways to harvest the oil that is used in medicine, food production, and beauty products throughout the world. The "all-wet process" uses raw coconut and is not commonly practiced. This method has drawbacks that include keeping the wet mash that is created from spoiling. The most widely practiced process involves using dried coconut kernel, or copra, to create oil that is "RBD", which stands for "refined, bleached, and deodorized." The kernel is placed in a hot press that, when applied, produces the precious oil. RBD oil is completely tasteless and odorless. It is the type of oil used in beauty products. Because coconut oil consists of a very small molecular structure, it is easy for our skin and hair to absorb. It is an absolutely perfect moisturizer that offers the added benefit of natural antibacterial and anti-fungal agents. So, it can serve a dual purpose: beautifying and protecting!

What Should I Look for When Purchasing Coconut Oil?

You can find many options for coconut oil on the Internet or in health food stores. Many larger grocery chains have expanded their inventory to include specialized sections that offer organic and natural options, so this may be a usable source, too. Coconut oil will come in a jar and will be in solid form like butter or shortening. You will find, however, that coconut oil melts at a lower temperature than other solid oils. Even in its solid form, it is pliable and soft.

Finding the right oil to use for beauty and hair care should not be difficult. You can leave behind the notion that the word "virgin" added to the beginning of coconut oil has implications regarding the quality of the oil as it does with olive oil. When it comes to coconut oil, the term does not hold particular relevance. Search for a refined oil as it will be fragrance free. You will find that the fragrance free variety is preferable, unless you happen to be head-over-heels in love with the smell of coconut. People with sensitivities to smells may not react well to unrefined oil and its ever present scent. Also, strongly scented oil may not blend well with other ingredients you may want to mix with it. Selecting a refined and scentless variety is a safer bet.

Your selection of coconut oil should depend upon your personal budget. The beauty benefits and effectiveness of the oil will not vary greatly between a highly marketed, sleekly packaged variety and a less prettily presented package, so this is one cosmetic that does not necessarily improve with cost.

There are a few basic things that you should consider when purchasing coconut oil. It should be white when in solid form and clear when heated. If the appearance is any other than this, do not purchase the oil. It may be contaminated or fake. Also, you may want to consider buying coconut oil in bulk to save money. It can get expensive when purchased in smaller amounts. It has a 12 month shelf-life, so the oil will not spoil quickly if you have extra on hand.

Using Coconut Oil Magic for Your Hair Care Needs

The hair that grows from our skin's pores requires care just like the rest of our body does. Coconut oil can offer help for a multitude of issues from medical issues of the scalp to the daily wear and tear you put on your hair through the use of product and heat.

The masks that will follow involve adding at least one ingredient to coconut oil, but we should first look at how coconut oil can help your hair on its own.

- Coating your hair with coconut oil 15 minutes before you get in the shower will "pre-shampoo" your hair. By opening up the follicles of your hair, it allows the shampoo and conditioner you normally use to work more effectively.
- People with coarse textured or curly hair have found coconut oil to work wonders to keep their hair smooth and manageable when used as a leave-in conditioner. If your hair is frizzy, a small amount of coconut oil worked into the bottom half and ends will help to control frizzy, flyaway hair.
- Medium textured hair responds well to the application of coconut oil left in overnight, but should be rinsed clean in the morning.
- Hair that is fine textured can benefit from short term application that is shampooed afterward.
- If your hair is naturally oily, you should use the oil for shorter times and avoid applying it directly to your scalp. Do not use the oil as a leave-in conditioner; rinse it completely out after about 10 minutes.

- While naturally oily hair can reap the benefits of coconut oil masks, it may prove more difficult to wash mask out of your hair. Following the lather, rinse, and repeat method, using a small amount of Dawn dishwashing soap as shampoo, will take the weighty residue out of your hair.
- Coconut oil applied directly to your hair can provide protection from the sun and its drying rays. If you are headed to the beach or any other sunny spot, a good coating of coconut oil forms a protective layer that keeps your hair from being damaged. It also gives your hair added resiliency that helps stop breakage and split ends that plague dried out hair.
- Used alone, coconut oil can also be used quite effectively as a styling product. Once the warm oil has a chance to cool on the hair, it returns to its solid form, reinforcing your hair's ability to hold style while retaining its bounce and shine.

Coconut Oil Hair Masks that Help with Scalp and Hair Problems

Here are some coconut oil mask recipes created with other added ingredients. The suggested length of the treatment is included with each mask, but you may find it necessary to adjust the time according to unique characteristics and needs of your hair.

Coconut Oil Masks to Control Dandruff

1: Coconut Oil and Gooseberry Mask

Using a combination of coconut oil and gooseberry juice will control any dandruff issue. Gooseberry trees can be found in many areas. Picking your own would be the inexpensive route, although the fruit can also be found in health food stores. Studies into the cause of dandruff have shown it to be caused by a contracted fungus. The anti-fungal properties of coconut oil tackle this issue head-on.

Ingredients:

Gooseberry Juice - 1 tbsp

Coconut Oil – 2 tbsp

Directions:

To obtain the juice you must grate the berries. Press the juice from the grated fruit, collecting it in a small pan. Once you have collected about 1 tablespoon of juice, add about 2 tablespoons of coconut oil. Place in a double boiler over hot water, not boiling, until the coconut oil melts. Mix well and apply thoroughly to your scalp, massaging in with your fingertips. Leave on your scalp for 1 hour and rinse. This natural remedy avoids medicinal shampoos and is just as effective for controlling the itching and flaking of annoying dandruff.

2: Coconut/Sesame Oil Mask

Another home remedy for dandruff control can be prepared by mixing coconut oil with sesame oil in equal parts.

Ingredients:

1 Cup coconut oil

1 Cup sesame oil

Directions:

Warm the oils until the coconut oil melts. Apply this mixture to your entire scalp and leave on for about 30 minutes. Shampoo as you normally would. This mask costs a fraction of shampoos designed to treat dandruff.

3: Peppermint Mask

This mask works wonders to help an oily scalp that produces dandruff.

Ingredients:

Coconut Oil – 3 tbsp

Peppermint Oil – 12- 15 drops

Directions:

Warm about 3 tablespoons of coconut oil until it has melted and add 12-15 drops of peppermint oil. Mix the two well and apply liberally to your scalp and to the first 3 or 4 inches of your hair.

4: Coconut Oil, Tea Tree & Rosemary

This mask is for dandruff-prone, flaky, dry or acne-ridden scalps.

Ingredients:

Coconut Oil – 6 tbsp

Jojoba Oil – 6 tbsp

Rosemary Oil – 3-4 drops

Tea Tree Oil – 3-4 drops

Directions:

Mix 6 tbsp of organic coconut oil and jojoba or olive oil well. Mix with 4-6 drops of rosemary oil and 3-4 drops of tea tree oil. Apply this mask on your scalp, running with your fingers in circular motion for 15 minutes. Leave it for 20 minutes. Then, wash your hair with your regular shampoo. Finish with a good conditioner.

5: Coconut Oil, Lemon Juice and Grapefruit Juice

This mask is for oily scalp. It rebalances the scalp oil and hydration levels. It removes toxins from scalp, calms down the sensitive skin and stimulates hair follicle growth.

Ingredients:

Coconut Oil – 6 tbsp

Grapefruit Juice – 2 tbsp

Lemon Juice – 3 tbsp

Directions:

Mix 6 tablespoon of organic coconut oil with 2 tbsp of grapefruit juice and 3 tbsp of lemon juice. Apply this mixture on your scalp with the help of hair dye brush or you can use a cotton ball. Make sure mixture is evenly distributed. Then gently massage your scalp for 10 – 15 minutes. Leave the mixture for 20 minutes and then wash with your regular shampoo. Finish with a good conditioner.

6: Coconut Oil with Honey and Apple Cider Vinegar

This mask is highly effective for various scalp problems, such as itchy scalp, dandruff, etc. ACV balances the natural pH of your hair. It removes buildup from hair styling products. It also makes your hair shiny and smooth.

Ingredients:

Coconut Oil - 2 Parts

Apple Cider Vinegar (ACV) - 1 Part

Raw Honey – 2 Parts

Directions:

Mix all these ingredients together. Apply this mask to wet or dry hair. Comb through with your fingers. Give your scalp and hair a gentle massage. Let sit for 30 minutes with heat or an hour without heat. Wash it off with your regular shampoo and finish with conditioner.

7: Coconut Oil with Aloe Vera

This hair mask is best home remedy for dandruff, itchy and dry scalp. Aloe vera has anti-fungal and anti-bacterial properties. It also helps control hair fall. For best results, you can use this mask twice a week. However, it is strongly recommended to do a patch test before using this mask on your hair. This is because aloe vera doesn't suit some people.

Ingredients:

Aloe Vera – 2 Medium-sized stems

Coconut Oil

Directions:

Take 2 medium-sized stems of aloe vera and extract the gel. Then, add in equal quantity of coconut oil. Make sure you use pure coconut oil without any artificial fragrances or additives. Blend this mixture well using your fingers. Apply this mask to your scalp and hair. Make sure you cover your hair from root to tip. Let sit for 30 minutes and then wash it off with lukewarm water. Then, wash with a mild shampoo (preferably sodium free).

Coconut Oil Masks to Slow Balding and Hair Loss and to Stimulate Hair Growth

8: Coconut Oil with Cinnamon and Honey

This mask contains cinnamon which stimulates hair growth by improving blood circulation in your scalp. Honey helps prevent hair from breakage. Coconut oil locks the moisture into your hair. It prevents protein loss from both damaged and undamaged hair.

Ingredients:

Cinnamon – 1 tsp

Organic Honey – 1 tbsp

Coconut Oil – 1 tbsp

Plain Yogurt – 1/2 tbsp

Directions:

In a bowl, add in the cinnamon, yogurt and honey first. Mix these ingredients well. You can use melted or solid coconut oil. Mix all these ingredients well. Apply this mask to your scalp and hair. Give your scalp a gentle massage. You can also apply this mask from roots to the ends. Leave this mask for about 1.5 hours. Wash your hair with your regular shampoo.

9: Coconut Oil and Lemon Juice Mask

Coconut oil has proven effective in stimulating hair growth even in places that have already become bald. It strengthens the hair follicles and encourages growth in those who suffer from alopecia. It also helps chemotherapy patients re-grow a head of healthy hair after losing it all during treatment.

Ingredients:

Coconut Oil – 2 Parts

Lemon Juice – 1 Part

Directions:

Take 2 parts of coconut oil and mix it in 1 part lemon juice. After warming and stirring well, apply this mixture to your scalp and hair from the scalp to the very tips. Take care to apply liberally to thinning or bald areas. Cover head with a shower cap and leave on at least 4 hours. The treatment is most effective if left on overnight.

10: Coconut Oil and Banana Mask

This vitamin-filled mask stimulates hair growth and makes existing hair stronger. It helps prevent hair loss.

Ingredients:

Banana – 1

Coconut Oil – 1 tbsp

Coconut Milk – 2 tbsp

Honey – 2 tbsp

Directions:

Put a sliced banana, 1 tablespoon of coconut oil, 2 tablespoons of coconut milk, and 2 tablespoons of honey into a blender and whip until the mixture reaches a fluffy consistency. Apply to your scalp and your hair. Leave the mask on your hair for 40 minutes then rinse well with lukewarm water.

11: Stimulating Sage Scalp Mask

Sage stimulates hair growth through improving the overall health of your scalp. It also works at the scalp level to stop hair loss.

Ingredients:

Coconut Oil – 3 tbsp

Sage Leaves (fresh or dried) – 6 – 7

Directions:

Place about 3 tablespoons of coconut oil in a small pan and add 6 or 7 fresh or dried sage leaves. Fresh leaves are more powerful, but dried ones are effective, too. Heat the oil and leaves to boiling then remove from the heat and cover. Let the mask cool enough to apply, and then massage the mixture into your scalp only.

12: Castor & Coconut Oil Mask

This mask stimulates hair growth. It also stops hair fall. It is also used to add volume to your hair. It will make your hair shiny and thick.

Ingredients:

Castor Oil – 5 tbsp

Coconut Oil – 5 tbsp

Directions:

Combine 5 tablespoons of castor oil and 5 tablespoons of coconut oil. Hair should be dry when applying this mask. Massage into the scalp for about five minutes. Then cover the rest of your hair. Leave the mask on for at least 3 hours. Letting it work overnight brings better results. Rinse and shampoo well to remove the oils. Using this mask a few times a week for a couple months will greatly increase your hair's growth rate.

13: Coconut Oil & Your Regular Shampoo

This mask moisturizes dry scalp and hair. It also stimulates hair growth.

Ingredients:

Your Regular Shampoo (Preferably Sodium Free)

Coconut Oil

Directions:

Take your regular shampoo and mix it with coconut oil in same quantity. Apply the shampoo to your hair by thoroughly mixing it. Wash your hair normally. Pat dry your hair.

14: Coconut Oil with Almond Oil

This mask promotes hair follicle growth. It helps to get rid of hair loss.

Ingredients:

Coconut Oil

Almond Oil – Few Drops

Directions:

Take sufficient amount of coconut oil and add few drops of almond oil. Mix them well until combined. Massage this mask on your scalp for about 10 – 15 minutes. Then leave it for about an hour. Wash it off with sodium free shampoo.

15: Coconut Oil with Essential Oils

This mask helps to get rid of hair loss problem. It stimulates hair re-growth.

Ingredients:

Essential Oil (Rosemary/Ylang Ylang/Peppermint/Lavender Oil/Basil Oil) – Few Drops

Coconut Oil – 1 Cup

Directions:

Take a jar of coconut oil. If it's solid, melt it in a water bath over lower heat. Take a cup of melted organic coconut oil and add few drops of either basil oil, lavender oil, rosemary oil, ylang ylang oil or peppermint oil. Mix this mixture well and pour it into a bowl. Take a few tbsp of this mixture and apply it on your dry hair. Them, comb it thoroughly. Cover your head with a shower cap or a wet towel. Leave it on your scalp for about 2 – 3 hours. You can also leave it overnight for best results. Rinse it off with regular shampoo and finish with conditioner. You can use this mask once a week to get rid of hair loss problem.

16: Coconut Oil and Shana Seeds

This is another powerful coconut oil mask to stop hair fall and to stimulate hair growth.

Ingredients:

Coconut Oil

Shana Seeds

Essential Oil of Your Choice

Directions:

Mix coconut oil with any essential oil of your choice (my personal favorite is ylang ylang and rosemary), and the powder of shana seeds. Make a fine paste by mixing these ingredients. Then put it on your scalp on regular basis. Leave this paste on your scalp for about 15 to 20 minutes. Rinse it off thoroughly.

17: Coconut Oil with Mustard

This hair mask has the power of mustard which works wonders for hair growth. This mask is also very helpful in stopping hair loss.

Warning: Mustard is a very strong irritating ingredient. It can cause allergic reaction on sensitive scalp and open sores. It is strongly recommended to do a patch test before using this mask. For a patch test, dilute a pinch of mustard powder in a drop of water and apply it on your neck. If your skin is slightly burning, it indicates a normal reaction. If you feel itching or if your skin looks ugly, mustard mask is not the right option for you and you should avoid using this mask. Also, don't get the mustard in your eye during application and washing off. Mustard can have a drying effect on your hair. To avoid this, you can prepare your hair for this mask by warming up 3 tbsp of coconut oil and applying it to the length of your dry and unshampooed hair.

Ingredients:

Ground Mustard Powder – 2 tbsp

Warm Water – 3 – 4 tbsp

Egg Yolk – 1

Sugar – 1 – 2 tbsp (optional)

Coconut Oil – 1 tbsp

Directions:

Add mustard powder and hot water in a bowl. Then add the egg yolk and coconut oil to mustard paste and mix well. Make sure mask is not too thick or thin. Apply this mask onto your scalp, avoiding your hair as much as possible. Cover your scalp with a shower cap and leave the mask onto your scalp for 15 minutes. If you don't feel heat, you can add sugar to this mask next time. It is recommended to avoid sugar in the first application. Wash this mask off with lukewarm water. Make sure your eyes are protected. Shampoo and condition your hair as normal.

Coconut Oil Masks for Effective Natural Head Lice Removal

18: Vinegar & Coconut Oil Mask

For a method of head lice treatment that is more effective than the harsh over-the-counter types, you'll need a jar of coconut oil and a bottle of apple wine vinegar. If you are treating a child, these totally natural products are much safer than chemicals found in traditional solutions used to treat lice. First, rinse your hair with the vinegar, don't wash it out, but leave it in until the hair is dry. The vinegar works by dissolving the sticky substance that causes lice eggs to cling to your hair. Apply coconut oil to dry hair making sure to work it into the scalp and the entire length of your hair. Place a snug shower cap on your head and leave in place for about 8 hours. This gives the oil plenty of time to smother and kill the lice. After removing the shower cap, comb meticulously through hair with a fine-toothed comb to remove dead lice and loosened eggs. One application will take care of the issue and your hair will be deep conditioned as well!

Note: Using coconut oil as a leave in conditioner or styling product guards you against contracting head lice, too. The slick and smooth shafts of hair covered by coconut oil offer logistical problems for parasites that try to form an attachment.

19: Coconut Oil with Garlic

This mask has garlic which has antiseptic properties. It has strong fragrance which kills lice by suffocating them.

Ingredients:

Coconut Oil – 2-3 tbsp

Garlic – 10 cloves

Directions:

Grind 8 – 10 garlic into paste. Mix 2 – 3 tbsp of coconut oil with garlic paste. Apply this mask on your scalp and hair. Make sure you don't leave any part of your hair. Leave it on the scalp for about 30 minutes. Wash your hair with hot water. You can apply this mask regularly until you get rid of head lice.

20: Coconut Oil, Garlic & Green Tea

The fatty content of coconut oil suffocates the head lice and makes it difficult for them to maintain grip on the hair strands. The lubricating nature of coconut oil makes it difficult for head lice to move freely. It also prevents these parasites from multiplying.

Ingredients:

Fresh Garlic Extract – Few Drops

Lemon Extract – Few Drops

Green Tea – Few Drops

Coconut Oil – 3 tbsp

Directions:

Take few drops of fresh garlic extract, lemon extract, coconut oil and green tea. Mix these ingredients together to make a fine solution. Then coat your hair with this solution. Cover your scalp and hair with a towel or shower cap. Leave it for about 30 minutes and then rinse it off with your regular shampoo. Use this mask once a week for 2 months for best results.

21: Coconut Oil with Oregano Oil

Oregano has powerful anti-parasitic properties. It kills head lice.

Ingredients:

Oregano – 1 Part

Coconut Oil – 5 Parts

Directions:

Take 1 part of oregano oil and mix it with 5 parts of coconut oil. Mix it well and make sure oregano oil is properly diluted with coconut oil. Apply it to your scalp and hair, and leave it for 2 – 3 hours. Then, comb your hair and wash it off with regular shampoo. Repeat this process on a regular basis to get rid of head lice.

22: Coconut Oil with Tea Tree Oil

Tea tree oil, used alone or with coconut oil (or other products), can remove head lice.

Ingredients:

Coconut Oil – 2 tbsp

Tea Tree Oil – 3 – 5 Drops

Directions:

Take tea tree oil and mix it with coconut oil to form a mask. Apply this mask completely onto your scalp and hair. Then cover your scalp and hair with a shower cap or plastic bag. Leave it for 12 hours or overnight. Warm your hair either by using a hair dryer or sitting in the sunlight until the plastic bag feels warm to touch. Remove plastic bag after 12 hours and apply about 6 oz of shampoo directly onto your scalp without wetting it first. Give your hair a gentle massage and again cover your hair and scalp with a shower cap. Leave your hair for 30 minutes. Rinse your hair thoroughly and use a lice removal comb to comb from roots to ends. This will remove nits from your hair. After combing, rinse your hair again in order to remove remaining oil.

Coconut Oil Masks to Moisturize and Repair Dry and Damaged Hair

23: Coconut Oil and Honey

Honey and coconut oil can make a significant difference in keeping your hair in good health. Honey has synergistic effects on hair. Honey and coconut oil makes hair soft, more voluminous, and reduces frizz and premature graying of hair. They also have anti-fungal and anti-bacterial properties that help fight and prevent dandruff, along with other scalp issues.

Ingredients:

Coconut Oil – 1 Part

Raw Honey – 1 Part

Directions:

Mix equal parts coconut oil and raw honey, making enough mixture to sufficiently cover your hair. Heat the mixture slightly in a small sauce pan. You can apply the mask to your wet or dry hair. Application may be slightly easier with wet hair. Divide your hair into sections and methodically apply the warm mask to all of your hair. Cover head with a shower cap and leave in place for about 40 minutes. Rinse the mask from your hair and shampoo as usual.

24: Coconut Oil and Olive Oil Mask

Coconut oil with olive oil promotes healthy hair. Both oils fight dryness. Coconut oil prevents frizz and locks moisture in hair. It also protects hair from protein loss. This mask will moisturize your scalp and discourage flakes.

Ingredients:

Olive Oil – 1 Part

Coconut Oil – 2 Parts

Directions:

Combine 2 parts coconut oil with 1 part olive oil to make enough mask to cover the length of your hair. Apply the mixture to your hair, focusing on the dry ends. Cover your head with a shower cap and leave on the 15-30 minutes. Rinse and shampoo as usual.

25: Egg Yolk Mask

Egg yolk is full of proteins. It conditions your hair and enhances hair growth. It helps in rebuilding damaged hair by filling in weakened spots along the hair strand. Egg yolk infuses hair with moisture and is a perfect remedy for dry and damaged hair.

Ingredients:

Egg Yolk - 2

Coconut Oil – 2 tbsp

Water – 1/2 Cup

Directions:

Mix 2 egg yolks with 2 tablespoons of melted coconut oil. Dilute the mixture with 1/2 cup of water. Slowly and thoroughly apply to scalp and hair. After the mask has been on your hair for 20 minutes, rinse it well. Shampooing is not necessary.

Note: Egg is the perfect source of protein your hair needs, but using egg masks on your hair too often can cause it to become brittle and prone to breakage. However, used once or twice a month, this mask can keep your hair looking moisturized and healthy.

26: Avocado Frizzy Fix

Avocadoes prevent hair loss and promote hair growth. Avocadoes also help in improving the condition of hair by acting as a moisturizer for dry and damaged hair.

Ingredients:

Coconut Oil

Milk

Avocado – 1 Ripe

Directions:

You'll need coconut oil, milk, and 1 ripe avocado to prepare this mask. Peel the avocado and cut into chunks. Put into a blender or food processor and puree. Add the milk and melted oil to the puree and mix it well. Apply to cover your hair completely. Leave on for 20 minutes, then rinse well. Shampoo your hair to be sure avocado is removed.

27: Rosemary and Lavender Moisturizing Mask

This mask deeply moisturizes dry locks and also makes your hair smell fantastic!

Ingredients:

Coconut Oil – 1/4 Cup

Lavender Oil 10 – 15 Drops

Rosemary Oil – 10 – 15 Drops

Directions:

The essential oils used in this fragrant hair mask can be purchased online or found in health food stores. Combine 1/4 cup of coconut oil and 10 to 15 drops each of Lavender oil and Rosemary oil. Place in a lidded jar and store until the coconut oil has melted. Apply to your hair starting at the scalp. Work through to the ends. Leave the mask on your hair overnight and rinse the mask thoroughly in the morning before shampooing as usual. You can use this mask as frequently as you wish.

28: Nourishing Hair Oil Mask

This mask is packed with the hydrating power of olive oil, coconut oil and honey.

Ingredients:

Olive Oil – 2 tbsp

Coconut Oil – 1 tbsp

Honey – 1 tbsp

Epsom Salt – 1tsp

Directions:

Combine 2 tablespoons of olive oil, 1 tablespoon of coconut oil (melted), 1 tablespoon of honey, and 1 teaspoon of epsom salts in a blender. When mixture is smooth, the epsom salt may still be gritty. It will dissolve into your hair once you apply the mask to your hair. Once you have covered all of your hair, cover your head with a shower cap and leave on for 30 minutes. Rinse out the mask and shampoo hair as usual.

29: Coconut Oil, Eggs and Raw Honey

This mask helps lock moisture in dry hair. It keeps your hair hydrated. It is helps prevent dandruff and dryness.

Ingredients:

Coconut Oil – 2 tbsp

Raw Honey – 1 tbsp

1 Large Egg Yolk

Directions:

Take 2 tbsp of coconut oil, 2 tbsp of raw honey and 1 large egg yolk. If coconut oil is solid, heat it over low heat until it melts. Then, remove it from heat and whisk in raw honey. Whisk for a minute or two to mix them properly. In a bowl, gently whisk the egg yolk (or you can take the whole egg if you prefer). Then slowly add in the raw honey and coconut oil mixture. Whisk these ingredients to combine. Apply to dry hair and scalp. Gently massage into your hair and the scalp. Make sure your entire scalp is covered with this mixture. Cover your hair with a shower cap and leave this mask on as long as you can. You can even leave it overnight. Squish your hair around every now and then through the shower cap. Rinse it with warm water until this mask is removed. You can apply gentle shampoo if you think your hair is still too oily.

30: Coconut Oil with Yogurt

Honey is a natural humectant. It retains moisture in your hair. It softens and smoothens your hair. It is rich in vitamins. Yogurt is rich in protein. It provides nourishment to your hair and stimulates growth. It is the best natural conditioner for hair. This mask will restore and maintain the natural look and health of your hair.

Ingredients:

Natural Yogurt – 2 tbsp

Honey – 1 tbsp

Coconut Oil – 1/4 tsp for thin hair, 1/2 tsp for thicker hair

Directions:

Melt coconut oil if it's solid, and then mix all ingredients well to form a paste. Apply this mask onto your hair, from the scalp to the ends. Gently massage your scalp for about 5 minutes. Leave the mask for 20 minutes. Wash your hair as normal. You can use this mask once a week.

31: Coconut Oil with Olive Oil, Egg and Banana

This is an excellent mask or dry and damaged hair. It is packed with the hydrating power of olive oil, banana and coconut oil. It will bring life to your hair by giving it a vitamin dose. Vitamin A, B, C, natural oils and carbohydrates in banana will help prevent split ends and breakage by improving the elasticity of your hair.

Ingredients:

Olive Oil – 2 tbsp

Egg – 1

Mayonnaise – 1 tbsp

Banana – 1

Honey – 1 1/2

Coconut Oil – 2 tbsp

Directions:

Add all ingredients in a food processor or blender and mix until smooth. Make sure there are no chunks in the paste. First rinse your hair with warm water and pat dry to remove excess liquid. Do not apply this mask on dry hair. Apply this mask from roots to ends. Gently massage into your scalp for a few minutes. Cover your head with a shower cap and leave the mask for 60 minutes. Wash your hair with cool water and pat dry. Warm a small amount of coconut oil in your hand and coat your hair. It will lock moisture and nutrients in your hair. You can use it either weekly or biweekly.

32: Coconut Oil with Fish Oil Capsules

Fish oil is rich in natural omega-3 and 6 oils that will stop split ends.

Ingredients:

Coconut Oil – 1 Spoon

Fish Oil Capsule – 2

Vitamin E Capsule – 2

Aloe Vera Gel – 1 Spoon

Castor Oil – 1/2 Spoon

Directions:

Squeeze the oil from vitamin E and fish oil capsules in an empty container. Add castor oil and coconut oil in that container. Mix aloe vera gel with these oils well. Apply this mask on damp hair and leave for an hour. Wash your hair with your regular shampoo. Finish with conditioner.

33: Coconut Oil with Vitamin E

This mask will deep condition, nourish and cleanse your scalp and hair.

Ingredients:

Coconut Oil

Sweet Almond Oil

Jojoba Oil

Olive Oil

Vitamin E Capsules – 3

Directions:

Mix all these oils together with vitamin E in equal amount. Massage this mask onto your scalp for 10 minutes and then leave overnight for best results. You can use this mask on every alternative day for maximum benefit.

34: Coconut Oil with Sunflower Oil

This mask is highly effective to restore moisture to your scalp and hair. It strengthens and repair damaged hair. It stimulates hair growth and controls frizz.

Ingredients:

Sunflower Oil – 1tbsp

Coconut Oil – 1 tbsp

Lavender Oil – 3 – 4 Drops

Directions:

Warm sunflower and coconut oil over lover heat until melted. Add in 3-4 drops of lavender oil. Apply this mask on the roots slowly. Make sure your roots are fully covered. Then, comb through your hair so all your hair gets coated in this mask. Leave it onto the scalp for 2 hours and then rinse out. You can also leave it overnight and wash your hair with a sodium (SLS) free shampoo. You can use this mask 2-3 times per week for 1-2 months.

Coconut Oil Masks to Brighten Dull Hair

35: Papaya & Yogurt Mask

Papaya is rich in vitamins and enzymes that give your hair nourishment while also cleaning off any build up.

Ingredients:

Papaya – 1

Coconut Oil – 2 tbsp

Plain Yogurt – 1/2 Cup

Directions:

Peel one papaya and remove the seeds. Put the papaya in a blender and add 2 tablespoons of melted coconut oil and 1/2 cup of plain yogurt. Apply to wet hair from the scalp to the ends and wrap tightly in a warm towel. After 30 minutes, shampoo hair as usual. By power cleaning dull hair, papaya uncovers its natural glow.

36: Mayonnaise Mega-shine Mask

Mayonnaise has long been known for its conditioning qualities, but it also adds a bright sheen to your hair.

Ingredients:

Mayonnaise – 1/2 Cup

Coconut Oil – 1/4 Cup

Egg Yolk – 1

Directions:

Mix together 1/2 cup of mayonnaise that has been set out to reach room temperature, 1/4 cup of warmed coconut oil and 1 large egg yolk. Apply the mask evenly to your hair then wrap it snugly in a towel for about 15 minutes. Rinse thoroughly with water only--do not shampoo your hair. Your hair might look a bit oily for a day, but the mask that remains will continue conditioning your hair. Wash your hair as usual the next day to remove any of the remaining mask. You will be impressed with the bright, healthy shine that this mask leaves behind.

37: Strawberry Mask

Strawberries promote hair growth, provide hydration, add a glossy shine and fight frizz for a while.

Ingredients:

Strawberries – 7

Coconut Oil – 1 tbsp

Honey – 1 tbsp

Directions:

Put about 7 strawberries, 1 tablespoon of coconut oil, and 1 tablespoon of honey into a blender and mix it to a puree. Apply the mask to hair thoroughly and leave on for about 30 minutes. Rinse well. Not only will strawberries give your hair extra shine, it also smells great.

38: Coconut Oil with Gelatin

Gelatin is full of protein, coconut oil moisturizes the scalp and hair, while olive oil acts as a natural conditioner. This mask is perfect to rejuvenate your dull hair.

Ingredients:

Coconut Oil – 3 tbsp

Olive Oil – 2 tbsp

Unflavored Gelatin – 2.5 tsp

Directions:

Mix all ingredients well in a small bowl. Apply this mask onto your scalp. Put a shower cap and leave it for 20 minutes. Shampoo and condition your hair as normal.

39: Coconut Oil with Avocado and Olive Oil – For Extra Shiny Hair

Avacado will make your super shiny. The coconut and olive in this mask will keep your hair hydrated.

Ingredients:

Avocado – 1 Ripe

Coconut Oil – 1/2 Cup

Olive Oil – 3 tsp

Directions:

Mash avocado with a spoon to make a smooth paste. Add coconut oil and olive oil. Mix these ingredients well. Warm this mask in a pre-heated pan for 20 seconds. Apply it to your hair from roots to ends. Gently massage it into your scalp. Leave it on the scalp for 30 minutes. Shampoo your hair as normal.

Coconut Oil Masks to Make Your Hair Extra Soft and Silky

40: Whipped Coconut & Jojoba Mask

Jojoba acts as a carrier for coconut oil in this treatment. It enhance coconut oil absorption into the scalp.

Ingredients:

Coconut Oil – 1/2 Cup

Jojoba Oil – 2 tbsp

Directions:

Melt 1/2 cup of coconut oil and add 2 tablespoons of Jojoba oil. Mix the two well with a whisk. Place the bowl of oil in the freezer for about 20 minutes. When you remove it, a hard top will have formed. Under the hardened oil you will find liquid oil. Using a hand mixer on low, cream the hardened and liquid oils to create a pasty substance. Spoon this into a jar with a lid and it will last for several applications. Work the mask through your entire head of hair and leave it on for about 10 minutes. Rinse and shampoo.

41: Coconut & Argan Oil Mask

Argan oil is often called 'liquid gold.' It is rich in many beneficial nutrients like vitamin E and fatty acids. It is a natural hair moisturizer. It makes hair soft, silky, and shiny. It also helps to treat split ends and control frizzy hair.

Ingredients:

Coconut Oil – 2 tbsp

Argan Oil – 10 drops

Directions:

Put 2 tablespoons of coconut oil and 10 drops of Argan oil into a small ziplock baggie and seal. Put the baggie under hot running water until the coconut oil has reached liquid form. Open the baggie and use your fingers to retrieve the oil and apply it to the full length of your hair. Then, comb the mask even through your hair and cover your head with a shower cap. Allow the mask to remain on your hair all night and shampoo out in the morning.

42: Maple & Coconut Mask

Maple syrup is a natural remedy for super dehydrated hair. It can bring life to your brittle hair.

Ingredients:

Maple Syrup – 1 Part

Coconut Oil – 1 Part

Directions:

This mask requires REAL maple syrup--not syrup that is maple-flavored. Combine equal parts of coconut oil and maple syrup and mix well to get all lumps smoothed out. Apply lavishly to your hair and cover with a towel. Leave on for about 1 hour, then shampoo and condition as usual.

43: Banana & Avocado Mask

This mask makes your hair easy to comb through and extremely soft.

Ingredients:

Banana – 1 Ripe

Coconut Oil – 2 tbsp

Avocado – 1 Ripe

Directions:

Use 1 ripe banana, 1 ripe avocado, and 2 tablespoons of melted coconut oil. Mix until smooth. Apply to hair and leave on for 30 minutes. Use regular shampoo to wash the mask out and condition as you normally would.

44: Coconut Oil with Mint

Mint stimulates hair follicles and blood circulation. It brightens dull hair by giving them a boost of energy. It also helps maintain natural pH balance of scalp. This way it controls excessive oil production.

Ingredients:

Coconut Oil

Rosemary Leaves (fresh or dried)

Mint Leaves (fresh or dried)

Directions:

Add unrefined, cold-pressed coconut oil in a sterile glass bottle. Add fresh or dried rosemary leaves and mint to the bottle. Make sure these herbs are fully dry. Seal the bottle and set in a warm spot for about 2 weeks. You can shake the bottle often to release essential oils. After 2 weeks, strain out the herbs and reserve your oil. You can use this oil for six months. Simply massage 2 tbsp of this oil onto your scalp and down to your ends. Leave it for about half an hour. Wash it off. You can use it once a week.

Coconut Oil Masks to Stop Grey Hair

45: Coconut Oil & Henna Mask

Henna is a wonderful natural hair colorant. It makes your hair darker. It strengths and conditions your hair.

Ingredients:

Henna Leaves – 12 Gram

Black Caraway – 7 Gram

Cloves – 2 Gram

Coconut Oil – 250 ml

Directions:

Add henna leaves, cloves, and black caraway to coconut oil and then warm them on lower heat until all these ingredients burnt. Then, preserve this oil into bottle and use every night before going to bed. Do thorough massage and apply it on the roots of hair. You can use this oil for a month and your hair will turn black.

46: Coconut Oil with Amla (Indian Gooseberry)

Amla is rich in antioxidants and vitamin C. These ingredients catalyze hair growth. Amla further prevents your hair from premature graying. Amla also helps revitalize the pigmentation in your hair. It cures grey hair problem.

Ingredients:

Indian Gooseberry (Amla) - 1 tsp

Fenugreek Powder – 1 tsp

Coconut Oil – 1 Cup

Directions:

Take teaspoon of amla powder and mix it with 1 teaspoon of fenugreek powder. Then add this mixture in a pan and add 1 cup coconut oil Heat this mixture on lower flame for few minutes until the oil turns brown. Allow it to cool for few minutes, but make sure it doesn't become solid. Strain the oil and store it in airtight, sterile jar. Apply this mask on to you scalp and hair, and massage gently. It is best to use it overnight. Wash it off in the morning. Apply this mask daily to get rid of grey hair.

47: Coconut Oil with Curry Leaves

Curry leaves are not only helpful for stopping hair loss, but also they are used to stop premature greying of hair. Curry leaves also revitalize dull hair. They make hair stronger and shinier.

Ingredients:

Handful Curry Leaves

Coconut Oil – 100ml

Directions:

Add a handful of curry leaves to 100 ml of coconut oil in a pan. Put it on stove over medium heat. Boil these ingredients together till the leaves turn black. Turn off the heat and strain the oil. Apply this oil on scalp and hair, and gently massage your scalp for about 15 – 20 minutes. Leave it overnight. Wash it off in the morning with your regular shampoo. You can use this mask every night for at least 3 months.

48: Coconut Oil with Ridge Gourd

Ridge gourd is commonly used to treat premature graying of the hair. It helps restore the natural pigment. It enhances hair roots.

Ingredients:

Dried Ridge Gourd – 1/2 Cup

Coconut Oil – 1 Cup

Directions:

Take 1/2 cup of dried ridge gourd and soak them in 1 cup of coconut oil for about 3 – 4 days. Then boil this mixture won low flame till oil gets darkened and becomes black. Strain the oil and store this to use for regular use. Apply this oil on scalp and massage gently for few minutes. Leave it for few hours or overnight for best results. Use it for at least 2 – 3 times per week till you get normal hair color.

49: Coconut Oil with Fenugreek

This mask is highly effective to stop premature graying of hair and hair fall. It stimulates hair growth and protects natural color of your hair.

Ingredients:

Fenugreek – 1 tsp

Coconut Oil – 2 tsp

Directions:

You can make Fenugreek paste at home. First soak Fenugreek seeds in water for 5 hours. Then grind soaked seeds by adding few drops of water. Add coconut oil in to this paste and mix it well. Apply this mask onto your scalp on affected areas. Leave it for 30 minutes. Wash your hair with your regular shampoo (preferably a sodium free shampoo).

50: Coconut Oil with Hibiscus Flower

This mask accelerates hair growth. It stops premature graying of hair. It also cures dandruff.

Ingredients:

Hibiscus Flower – few

Coconut Oil – 2 tbsp

Directions:

Mix hibiscus flowers with coconut oil to make a paste. Apply this paste onto your scalp and hair. Rinse it off thoroughly with a mild shampoo.

Hopefully, you have found some of these easy hair masks can be used to reach your beauty goals. None of the recipes require exotic or hard to find ingredients. Many of the nourishing items can probably be found in your kitchen right now. Instead of investing in costly hair repair treatments to repair damage, try a simple mask. Rather than buying medicated shampoos that are hard on your hair to treat your scalp issues, you might find that investing in a bottle of peppermint oil takes care of your problem for as long as six months. Why not try out this less expensive approach to see if it helps you achieve a head full of healthy, bouncy, shiny hair? Just zero in on the right coconut oil for your budget, pick up a jar, and take your hair treatment plan into your own hands.

Coconut Oil with Essential Oils

Did you know that you can use coconut oil with any essential oil of your choice? You can make your own homemade hair repair treatment just by adding 1/2 teaspoon of any essential oil in 1 cup of melted coconut oil. The choice of essential depends upon which essential oil is best for your hair. It mainly depends on what you need it to do.

Here are some common hair problems, with their corresponding essential oil solutions. You can choose these essential oils to add in the coconut oil based on the hair problem you have.

To Stimulate Hair Growth:

Basil, Lemongrass, Lemon, Tea Tree, Rosemary, Ylang Ylang

For Dry Itchy Scalp/Dandruff:

Lavender, Bay, Cedar wood, Chamomile, Eucalyptus, Clary Sage, Frankincense, Lemon, Myrrh, Sage, Rose, Tea Tree and Sandalwood

For Dry Hair:

Peppermint, Myrrh

For Extra Conditioning/Shine:

Lavender, Chamomile

For Hair Loss:

Cedar wood, Burdock, Thyme, Jojoba

How to Use Coconut Oil with Essential Oils?

Take 1/2 teaspoon any of these essential oils (1 or 2, avoid using all of them at the same time) and mix with 1 cup of coconut oil. Apply this mask onto your scalp and hair. Wrap your head in a wet towel or cover your head with a shower cap. Make sure this mask is well distributed onto your scalp. Let sit for a few hours (minimum 30 minutes). Wash it off with your regular shampoo and conditioner.

How to Remove Coconut Oil from Your Hair?

The ease of removing coconut oil from your scalp and hair depends on the type of your hair and shampoo. Some people have no difficulty in washing it out of their hair, while others wash their hair any times and still remain unable to remove it from their hair. If you also have difficulty to get this natural deep conditioner out of your hair, here are two methods for you.

1: No Poo Method

This method involves the use of baking soda as shampoo and apple cider vinegar as a conditioner. You can use 1 – 2 tablespoon of baking soda per wash. Simply rub it on your wet scalp, the rinse it off. For conditioning, dilute about 50/50 apple cider vinegar and water in a spray bottle. Spray a handful this mixture on your hair from roots to ends. Let sit for a few minutes, and then rinse.

2: Egg Wash Followed by Castile Soap

Egg wash has great benefits. It removes buildup from hair styling products. It cuts through oil & grease. It is full of proteins that strengthen and thicken hair. It has vitamin A, D, & E which make your hair shinier.

Take 1 egg with 2 tbsp of water and mix well. Apply this mask onto your scalp and hair, and massage gently. Leave for 10 minutes and rinse with lukewarm water. Avoid using hot water. After rinsing your hair, apply a teaspoon of castile soap and gently massage onto your scalp and hair. Then rinse it off.

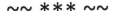

* * * *

Thank You from Ashley

Dear home-remedy enthusiast,, thank you for purchasing this
Coconut Oil for Hair homemade hair masks book.

From the Author

Ashley Frank

"I'm delighted to share my knowledge and advice about coconut oil
for hair. This is a subject I'm very enthusiastic about. It is my goal to
give women tips of the trade that will help them make their hair
look perfect, every day. In this book, I've shared 50 best coconut oil
hair masks that can be used to unlock the potential of your hair."

☙ Ashley ❧

* * * *

About Author

Ashley Frank is a writer and experienced cosmetologist. She is obsessed with everything related to hair. Her passion for hair and writing brought her to Kindle and Createspace. Ashley attends regular hair education shows and seminars to stay current on on-going trends and new techniques.

* * * *

References

Cover design: Angie

J Cosmet Sci. 2003 Mar-Apr;54(2):175-92. Effect of mineral oil, sunflower oil, and coconut oil on prevention of hair damage. Rele AS, Mohile RB. Research and Development Department, Nature Care Division, Marico Industries Ltd., Mumbai, India.

Printed in Great Britain
by Amazon